CHAIR YOGA FOR SENIORS LOSE BELLY FAT

Easy Stretches and Poses with Pictures That You Can Do Sitting Down at Home for Rapid Weight Loss and to Lose Belly Fat Very Fast. (Fitness for Seniors).

Jane Smith Adams

Copyright © 2023

All Rights Are Reserved

The content in this book may not be reproduced, duplicated, or transferred without the express written permission of the author or publisher. Under no circumstances will the publisher or author be held liable or legally responsible for any losses, expenditures, or damages incurred directly or indirectly as a consequence of the information included in this book.

Legal Remarks

Copyright protection applies to this publication. It is only intended for personal use. No piece of this work may be modified, distributed, sold, quoted, or paraphrased without the author's or publisher's consent.

Disclaimer Statement

Please keep in mind that the contents of this booklet are meant for educational and recreational purposes. Every effort has been made to offer accurate, up-to-date, reliable, and thorough information. There are, however, no stated or implied assurances of any kind. Readers understand that the author is providing competent counsel. The content in this book originates from several sources. Please seek the opinion of a competent professional before using any of the tactics outlined in this book. By reading this book, the reader agrees that the author will not be held accountable for any direct or indirect damages resulting from the use of the information contained therein, including, but not limited to, errors, omissions, or inaccuracies.

TABLE OF CONTENTS

INTRODUCTION

Understanding Chair Yoga: Benefits and Safety

Adapting Yoga for Accessibility and Comfort

Chair yoga reimagines traditional yoga by modifying poses to be performed while seated, or by using the chair as a support. This adaptation makes yoga accessible to those who might find standard yoga poses challenging, particularly seniors or individuals with limited mobility, balance issues, or chronic health conditions. By bringing yoga into a more accessible form, chair yoga opens up the world of yoga's benefits to a broader audience, ensuring that everyone, regardless of their physical capabilities, can partake in this enriching practice.

Enhancing Flexibility and Mobility

One of the most notable benefits of chair yoga for seniors is the improvement in flexibility and mobility. As we age, our joints and muscles tend to become less flexible, leading to stiffness and decreased range of motion. Chair yoga gently encourages movement in all the major joints and muscle groups, promoting flexibility and helping to alleviate stiffness. Regular practice can lead to greater ease in performing everyday activities, reducing the risk of falls and improving overall quality of life.

Improving Balance and Stability

Balance is a critical aspect of aging healthily, and chair yoga offers a safe way to improve it. The use of a chair provides stability, allowing practitioners to focus on the balance-enhancing aspects of yoga without the fear of falling. This can be particularly beneficial for seniors who are prone to balance issues, as improved balance is linked with a decreased risk of falls and related injuries.

Boosting Overall Wellness

Chair yoga isn't just about physical benefits; it also has a profound impact on overall wellness. The practice integrates breathing exercises and meditation, promoting mental clarity and stress reduction. For seniors, this can mean better sleep quality, improved mood, and a heightened sense of well-being. The meditative aspect of yoga helps in cultivating mindfulness, which can have positive effects on mental health, especially in combating feelings of isolation or depression that sometimes accompany aging.

Safety Guidelines and Personalization

Safety is paramount in chair yoga, especially for seniors with varying health concerns. This section of the book will provide detailed guidance on how to practice safely, including how to choose the right chair, how to modify poses to suit individual needs, and how to recognize one's own limits. We emphasize the importance of listening to one's body and making adjustments as needed. Special considerations will be given to common age-related conditions like osteoporosis, arthritis, and hypertension, ensuring that each reader can tailor their practice to their specific health requirements.

The Connection Between Yoga and Belly Fat Reduction

Holistic Impact on Health

Yoga is renowned for its holistic approach, harmonizing the body, mind, and spirit. In the context of belly fat reduction, this holistic approach is particularly beneficial. Chair yoga, a form of yoga adapted for those who may have difficulty with traditional poses, retains the core essence of yoga's holistic benefits. Regular practice can lead to improved physical health, enhanced mental clarity, and emotional balance.

Physical Benefits: Targeting Belly Fat

Chair yoga offers a series of movements and postures specifically designed to target the abdominal area. These poses often involve gentle twists, forward bends, and side stretches that engage the core muscles. Engaging these muscles is key to reducing belly fat. Additionally, many chair yoga poses help to improve overall body metabolism. An increased metabolic rate aids in burning calories more effectively, which is crucial in reducing fat accumulation, particularly around the abdomen.

Breathing Techniques: Enhancing Digestion and Metabolism

Breathing techniques, or pranayama, are an integral part of yoga. In chair yoga, these techniques are tailored to be accessible while seated. Deep, mindful breathing aids in stimulating the digestive system, thereby enhancing digestion and metabolism. A well-functioning digestive system is essential for the efficient processing of food and the prevention of fat accumulation in the body, especially in the abdominal area.

Stress Management: A Key Factor in Weight Control

Stress is a well-known contributor to weight gain, particularly in the abdominal region. Cortisol, a hormone released during stress, has been linked to increased belly fat. Yoga's emphasis on relaxation and mindfulness helps in managing stress and reducing cortisol levels. Chair yoga incorporates relaxation and meditation practices that are effective in calming the mind, thus indirectly assisting in the reduction of stress-induced belly fat.

Accessible and Sustainable Practice for Seniors

For seniors, the accessibility of chair yoga makes it a sustainable form of exercise. Regular practice is feasible and less intimidating, which is crucial for long-term adherence to any fitness regimen aimed at weight loss. By providing a form of exercise that is gentle yet effective, seniors are more likely to maintain a routine, leading to gradual and sustainable belly fat reduction.

Preparing for Chair Yoga: Equipment and Setting

Embarking on the journey of chair yoga requires more than just a willingness to start; it necessitates a thoughtful preparation of your physical space and the right equipment. This preparation is key to ensuring that your practice is both effective and enjoyable, paving the way for a transformative journey towards better health and reduced belly fat.

Choosing the Right Chair

The cornerstone of chair yoga is, unsurprisingly, the chair. Selecting the right chair can significantly impact your practice. The ideal chair is sturdy, without wheels, and has a flat seat that allows your feet to rest comfortably on the ground. The back of the chair should be straight to provide adequate support for your spine. Avoid chairs with arms, as they can restrict movement during various poses. If your feet don't comfortably reach the floor, consider using a cushion or a yoga block to elevate your sitting position.

Yoga Accessories

While the chair is the primary equipment, a few additional accessories can enhance your practice:

Yoga Mat: A mat provides a non-slip surface, essential for safety, especially if your chair is on a smooth floor.

Cushions and Pillows: These can be used for additional support and comfort, especially in poses that require extra cushioning for the back or knees.

Yoga Blocks: Blocks can be used to bring the ground closer to you in certain poses, aiding in alignment and stability.

Yoga Straps: Straps are helpful for those with limited flexibility, allowing you to safely perform stretches without straining.

Blankets: A folded blanket can be used for seated poses to elevate the hips and ensure a neutral spine position.

Creating a Conducive Environment

The physical space where you practice plays a crucial role in your yoga experience. Ideally, choose a quiet, well-ventilated area with enough room to move freely. Good lighting is essential; natural light is preferable, but if that's not possible, ensure your space is well-lit with artificial lighting. Minimize distractions by choosing a time when you're least likely to be disturbed, and consider turning off your phone or any other electronic devices.

Personalizing Your Space

Personalizing your yoga space can make your practice more enjoyable. Consider adding elements that calm your senses and help you focus:

Plants: Adding greenery can create a serene and natural environment.

Aromatherapy: Scented candles or essential oil diffusers with lavender or eucalyptus can enhance relaxation.

Soothing Music or Sounds: Gentle background music or nature sounds can help in creating a tranquil atmosphere.

Inspirational Items: Items like photographs, artwork, or small statues that inspire or calm you can be powerful additions.

Dress for Comfort and Movement

Wearing comfortable clothing that allows for unrestricted movement is crucial. Opt for breathable, stretchable fabrics that don't restrict your waist or limbs. Avoid belts, jewelry, or any accessories that could interfere with your movements or cause discomfort.

Safety Considerations

Safety should always be a priority. Ensure your chair is on a stable surface and won't slip during your practice. If you're using a yoga mat, check that it's free from tears or curls that could cause tripping. Keep the area around your chair clear of any obstacles or sharp objects.

Consistency in Practice

Having a dedicated space and time for your chair yoga practice can help establish a routine. Consistency is key to experiencing the full benefits of yoga, including weight loss and improved well-being. Try to practice at the same time each day to create a habit that becomes a natural part of your daily routine.

Mental Preparation

Finally, preparing your mind is as important as preparing your space. Before you begin each session, take a few moments to clear your mind and focus on your intentions for the practice. This mental preparation helps you stay present during your practice, enhancing the mind-body connection that is central to yoga.

CHAPTER 1

FUNDAMENTALS OF CHAIR YOGA FOR SENIORS

Chair yoga, a form of yoga modified to be more accessible for seniors, offers a myriad of benefits, making it an excellent practice for those seeking a gentle yet effective way to enhance their physical health and overall well-being. This comprehensive guide will delve into the fundamentals of chair yoga for seniors, covering essential aspects such as postures, breathing techniques, and warm-up exercises.

Introduction to Chair Yoga Postures

Chair yoga adapts traditional yoga poses to be performed while seated or using a chair for support. This adaptation makes yoga more accessible to seniors, particularly those with limited mobility or balance concerns. The beauty of chair yoga lies in its flexibility; it can be modified to suit various fitness levels and physical conditions.

Seated Mountain Pose (Tadasana):

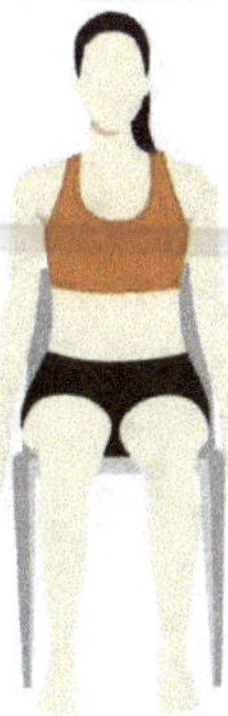

This foundational pose involves sitting upright with feet flat on the ground, hands resting on the knees or thighs. It helps in improving posture and spinal alignment.

Seated Cat-Cow Stretch: Involving the movement of the spine, this stretch enhances flexibility and relieves tension in the back and neck.

Chair Raised Hands Pose (Urdhva Hastasana):

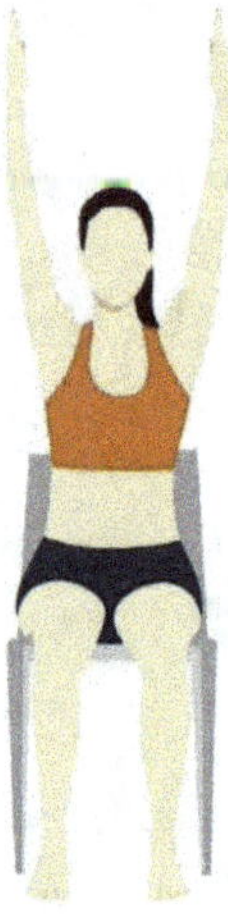

By extending the arms overhead, this pose aids in stretching the shoulders and improving upper body mobility.

Seated Forward Bend (Paschimottanasana):

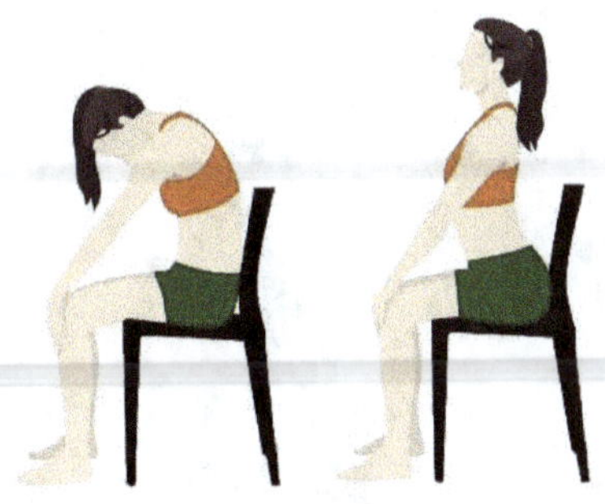

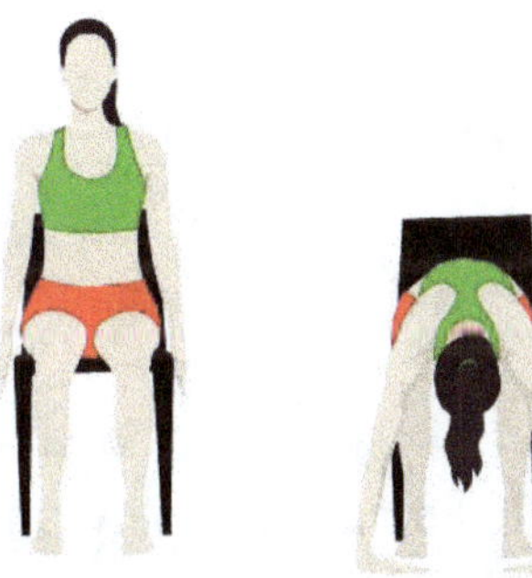

This pose stretches the back and legs, promoting flexibility and aiding in digestion.

Seated Twist (Ardha Matsyendrasana):

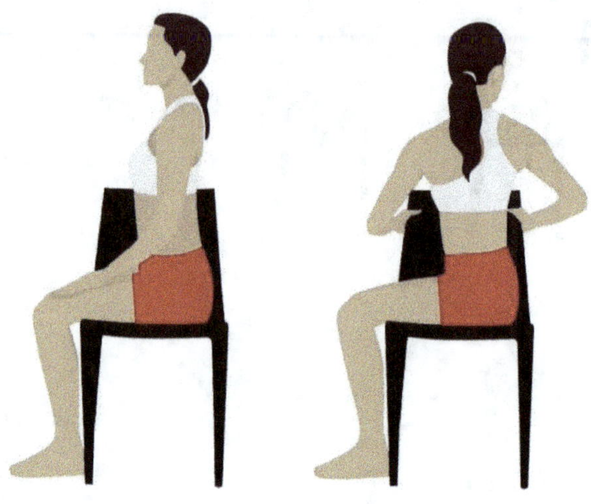

Twisting poses are excellent for spinal mobility and can aid in detoxifying the body.

Chair Warrior Pose:

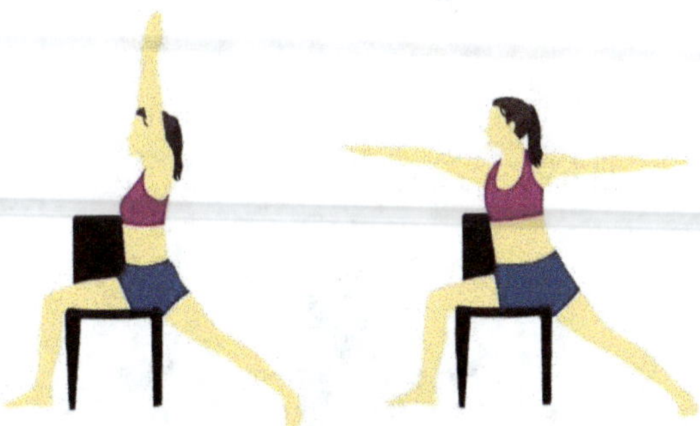

A gentle version of the classic warrior pose, it strengthens the legs and improves balance while seated.

Seated Tree Pose:

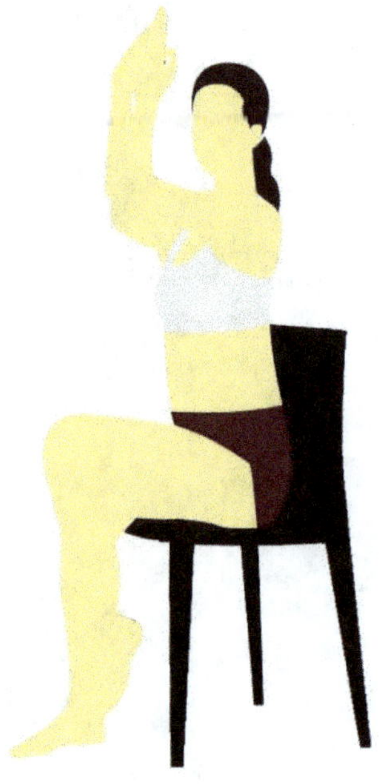

This pose helps in improving balance and stability and can be done either seated or using the chair for support.

These postures are not only beneficial for physical health but also for mental well-being, as they encourage mindfulness and a connection between the body and breath.

Breathing Techniques for Enhanced Yoga Practice

Breathing, an integral aspect of yoga, plays a crucial role in unifying the physical and mental components of the practice. In chair yoga, especially designed for seniors, mastering various breathing techniques can significantly amplify the benefits of the practice. These techniques enhance relaxation, improve lung capacity, and increase the flow of oxygen and energy, vital for both physical health and mental well-being. Let's delve into some key breathing techniques that can be seamlessly integrated into chair yoga.

Diaphragmatic Breathing (Belly Breathing)

Diaphragmatic breathing, commonly known as belly breathing, is a fundamental breathing technique in yoga. It involves deep breathing through the diaphragm rather than shallow breathing through the chest. This type of breathing is particularly beneficial for seniors as it promotes relaxation and stress reduction, crucial for maintaining a healthy mind and body at an older age.

How to Practice:

- Sit comfortably in your chair with your feet flat on the ground.
- Place one hand on your abdomen and the other on your chest.
- Breathe in slowly through your nose, feeling your abdomen expand under your hand.
- Exhale gently through your mouth or nose, feeling the abdomen fall.
- Repeat this process, focusing on the rise and fall of your abdomen.

This technique enhances lung capacity and oxygenates the blood, leading to better energy levels and improved organ function. It also triggers the body's relaxation response, reducing stress and anxiety.

Three-Part Breath (Dirga Pranayama)

Three-Part Breath, or Dirga Pranayama, is a deeply soothing breathing technique that enhances lung function and calms the mind. It involves dividing the breath into three distinct parts: the abdomen, diaphragm, and chest.

How to Practice:

- Begin by breathing into your abdomen, allowing it to expand fully.
- Continue inhaling into your diaphragm, noticing your ribs expand sideways.
- Complete the inhalation by filling the upper chest, lifting it slightly.
- Exhale in reverse order: chest falls, ribs contract, and abdomen sinks.

This breathing method is especially beneficial for seniors, as it ensures the full utilization of lung capacity, often underused due to shallow breathing habits. It also helps in calming the mind, reducing the symptoms of anxiety, and improving focus.

Equal Breathing (Sama Vritti)

Equal Breathing, or Sama Vritti, involves inhaling and exhaling for an equal count. This symmetry in breathing helps in focusing the mind, reducing anxiety, and creating a sense of balance and tranquility.

How to Practice:

- Sit in a relaxed posture with your spine straight.
- Inhale slowly and deeply to a count of four.
- Exhale to the same count of four.
- Continue this pattern, keeping the inhalation and exhalation equal.

This technique is particularly effective in chair yoga for seniors, as it can be practiced with ease and does not require physical exertion. It helps in centering the mind, leading to enhanced focus during yoga practice and everyday activities.

Alternate Nostril Breathing (Nadi Shodhana)

Alternate Nostril Breathing, or Nadi Shodhana, is a powerful technique that involves alternating the breath between the nostrils. This practice is said to balance the left and right hemispheres of the brain, resulting in mental clarity and stress relief.

How to Practice:

- Sit comfortably with your back straight.
- Place your left hand on your knee and your right hand in front of your face.

lose your right nostril with your right thumb and
hale slowly through the left nostril.

- Close the left nostril with your right ring finger, release the right nostril, and exhale slowly.
- Inhale through the right nostril, close it, and exhale through the left.

Continue this pattern for several cycles.

This breathing technique is particularly effective for seniors as it not only aids in mental clarity but also helps in regulating the body's cooling and heating mechanisms, which can be beneficial for those experiencing hormonal imbalances or stress-related symptoms.

Integrating Breathing Techniques into Chair Yoga Practice

Incorporating these breathing techniques into chair yoga practice can significantly enhance both the physical and mental benefits of the poses. For instance, practicing diaphragmatic breathing while engaging in a gentle seated twist can deepen the twist's effect and aid in relaxation. Similarly, using the three-part breath during a forward bend can enhance the sense of release and surrender in the pose.

Moreover, these breathing techniques can be practiced independently of the yoga poses, serving as standalone practices for stress relief, improved focus, or relaxation. They are particularly beneficial for seniors, as they can be practiced anywhere and at any time, requiring no special equipment or physical exertion.

Warm-Up Exercises: Preparing Your Body for Chair Yoga

Warm-up exercises are an essential component of any physical routine, particularly for seniors practicing chair yoga. These exercises are designed not just as a preliminary step but as a crucial part of the overall yoga experience. They serve multiple purposes: they prepare the body for more intensive movements, reduce the risk of injury, increase blood flow to the muscles, and help transition the mind from a state of rest to one of active engagement.

The Importance of Warm-Up Exercises

Before delving into the specific exercises, it's vital to understand why warm-ups hold such significance, especially for seniors. As we age, our muscles and joints become less flexible, and our response time slows down.

Warm-up exercises gently coax the body into a state of readiness, enhancing flexibility and reducing the likelihood of strains or sprains. They also stimulate blood flow, ensuring that muscles receive the oxygen and nutrients they need for the workout ahead. Additionally, warm-ups can be a meditative time to focus on the breath and prepare mentally for the yoga session.

Detailed Warm-Up Exercises for Chair Yoga

Neck Rolls

- **Purpose:** Neck rolls are a gentle way to release tension in the neck and shoulders, areas that often harbor stress.
- **How to Perform:** Sit upright in your chair with your feet flat on the ground. Drop your chin to your chest and gently roll your head in a circular motion. Do this slowly, feeling the stretch at each point of the circle. After a few rotations in one direction, switch and rotate in the opposite direction.
- **Benefits:** This exercise improves neck flexibility and can help alleviate headaches and stiffness.

Shoulder Shrugs and Circles

- **Purpose:** These movements help loosen the shoulders and upper back.
- **How to Perform:** Lift your shoulders up towards your ears, hold for a moment, and then release them down. Repeat this several times. For shoulder circles, lift your shoulders and then roll them back and down in a circular motion, and then reverse the direction.
- **Benefits:** They reduce tension and stiffness in the shoulder and neck area, and improve the range of motion.

Ankle and Wrist Rolls

- **Purpose:** Rotating the ankles and wrists helps to enhance joint mobility and circulation.
- **How to Perform:** Extend your legs and rotate your ankles in a circular motion. Do the same with your wrists, either holding them out or resting your forearms on your thighs.
- **Benefits:** These exercises are particularly beneficial for those with arthritis or stiffness in these joints.

Side Stretches

- **Purpose:** Side stretches help to open up the ribcage, enhancing lung capacity and improving posture.
- **How to Perform:** Raise one arm overhead and gently bend to the opposite side, keeping your arm close to your ear. Hold the stretch for a few breaths, then return to the center and repeat on the other side.
- **Benefits:** They not only stretch the sides of the body but also help in better breathing, which is crucial for yoga practice.

Gentle Spinal Twists

- **Purpose:** These are preparatory exercises for more intensive twisting poses, enhancing spinal mobility.
- **How to Perform:** Sitting upright, turn your upper body to one side, holding onto the back of the chair for support. Hold the twist for a few breaths before turning to the other side.

- **Benefits:** Spinal twists are excellent for maintaining spinal health, improving digestion, and relieving back pain.

Leg Extensions

- **Purpose:** Extending the legs helps in improving circulation and preparing the legs for more active poses.
- **How to Perform:** While seated, extend one leg at a time, pointing and flexing the foot. You can also perform small circular movements with the foot to enhance ankle mobility.
- **Benefits:** These movements help in preventing leg cramps and improving the strength and flexibility of the legs.

Incorporating Mindfulness into Warm-Ups

A unique aspect of warm-up exercises in yoga, including chair yoga, is the incorporation of mindfulness. As you perform these exercises, focus on your breath, aiming for deep, even inhalations and exhalations. This mindful approach not only prepares the body but also centers the mind, making the transition into yoga poses more fluid and focused.

Customizing Warm-Up Exercises

It's essential to listen to your body and modify these exercises as needed. Not every exercise will be suitable for every individual, and it's crucial to avoid any movements that cause pain or discomfort. Feel free to adjust the range of motion, the number of repetitions, or even skip certain exercises that don't suit your body.

"Warm-up exercises are not merely a preliminary step in the practice of chair yoga; they are a fundamental part of the experience, setting the tone for the session. They ensure that the body is adequately prepared for the yoga poses, thereby enhancing the effectiveness of the practice and minimizing the risk of injury. By integrating these exercises with a focus on mindful breathing and movement, seniors practicing chair yoga can maximize the benefits of their practice, ensuring a safe and enriching experience that nurtures both the body and mind."

CHAPTER 2

CHAIR YOGA ROUTINES FOR BELLY FAT REDUCTION

Core-Strengthening Chair Yoga Series

The Importance of a Strong Core

A strong core is vital for overall health and stability, particularly for seniors. It supports the spine, improves balance, and can help in reducing belly fat. Chair yoga offers a safe way to strengthen these muscles without the strain that floor exercises might cause.

Chair Yoga Exercises for Core Strengthening

- **Seated Mountain Pose with Core Engagement:** Sit erect with your feet flat on the ground. Inhale deeply and, as you exhale, engage your abdominal muscles by pulling your navel towards your spine. Hold this engagement for a few breaths, then release. Repeat several times.

- **Seated Marching:** Sit at the edge of the chair, spine straight. Slowly lift your right knee towards your chest, engaging your core, then lower it.

Repeat with the left knee. Alternate this marching motion for several rounds.

- **Chair Plank:** Sit forward on the chair, place your hands on the edges, and extend your legs out in front with heels on the ground. Lean forward slightly, keeping your body straight, to engage your core muscles. Hold this plank position for a few breaths.

Gentle Twists and Side Bends for Abdominal Toning

In the realm of chair yoga, gentle twists and side bends play a crucial role, especially when it comes to toning the abdominal area. These movements are not only beneficial for physical appearance but also for enhancing internal bodily functions like digestion. Let's delve deeper into these movements and explore their benefits, variations, and the proper techniques to perform them effectively.

Understanding the Benefits of Twists and Side Bends

1. **Enhancing Digestive Health:** Twists can stimulate the digestive organs, helping to improve

gut functionality. This stimulation aids in the detoxification process, potentially leading to improved metabolism and more efficient fat burning.

2. **Toning the Abdominal Muscles:** Regular practice of twists and bends can strengthen and tone the muscles in the abdominal area. This helps in creating a firmer, more sculpted waistline.

3. **Improving Flexibility and Range of Motion:** These movements can increase the flexibility of the spine and the sides of the body, contributing to overall mobility and balance, which are crucial for seniors.

4. **Stress Reduction:** Twists and bends can have a calming effect on the nervous system, aiding in stress reduction. Lower stress levels can contribute to reduced cortisol levels, which is beneficial for weight management.

Effective Chair Yoga Twists and Bends

1. Seated Spinal Twist

Technique: Sit sideways on the chair, ensuring your feet are flat on the ground. Hold onto the back of the chair with both hands for support. As you inhale, lengthen your spine, and as you exhale, gently twist your torso towards the back of the chair. Hold this position for a few breaths, feeling the twist elongate and energize your spine. Carefully switch sides to maintain balance in your body.

Variations and Tips: For a deeper twist, you can inhale to lengthen the spine further and then deepen the twist as you exhale. If twisting is challenging, simply hold the sides of the chair and twist to a comfortable degree.

2. Seated Side Bend

Technique: Sit with your feet firmly planted on the floor, spine erect. Inhale and raise your right arm overhead, and as you exhale, gently bend to the left. Keep your arm close to your ear, ensuring that the bend initiates from your waist, stretching the entire right side of your body. Hold for a few breaths, then inhale back to the center and switch sides.

Variations and Tips: If raising your arm overhead is difficult, rest your hand on your head for support. Ensure that you're bending from the waist and not compressing the opposite side. Keep your hips firmly on the chair to avoid tilting.

3. Seated Cat-Cow with a Twist

Technique: Sit with your feet flat and hands on your knees. Begin with the cat-cow stretch: inhale and arch your back slightly, lifting your chest and chin (cow), and as you exhale, round your back, tucking your chin to your chest (cat). Add a twist by gently turning to the right during the cat pose, then return to the center for the cow pose, and twist to the left during the next cat pose. Continue this sequence for several rounds.

Variations and Tips: Focus on synchronizing your breath with the movements, inhaling during the cow pose and exhaling during the cat pose and twists. The twist should be gentle and comfortable, without any strain.

Complementing Twists and Bends with Other Practices

To maximize the benefits of these exercises, it's beneficial to incorporate other elements of chair yoga and wellness practices:

1. **Breathing Exercises:** Pairing twists and bends with deep, mindful breathing can enhance their effectiveness, especially in terms of stress reduction and improving digestive functions.

2. **Core Strengthening Exercises:** Integrating core strengthening movements along with twists and bends can further tone the abdominal area and improve overall stability.

3. **Mindful Eating:** Complementing your yoga practice with a balanced diet can significantly impact your belly fat reduction efforts. Mindful eating encourages a healthier relationship with food, aiding in weight management.

4. **Regular Practice:** Consistency is key. Regular practice of these movements will yield better

results in terms of flexibility, muscle tone, and overall wellness.

Safety and Modifications

Always listen to your body and make modifications as necessary. Use props like cushions or yoga blocks for extra support, and avoid any movements that cause discomfort or pain. It's also advisable to consult with a healthcare provider before starting any new exercise regimen, especially if you have existing health conditions.

Chair Yoga Flow: Integrating Movement and Breath

Understanding the Importance of Breath in Chair Yoga

Before we dive into specific sequences, it's crucial to understand the role of breath in yoga. Breathing, in yoga, is not just a physical act of inhaling and exhaling; it's a bridge between the body and mind. When synchronized with movements, breathing can deepen the effectiveness of each pose, providing a more holistic benefit.

The Basics of Yogic Breathing

In yogic practice, the breath is often deep and controlled, originating from the diaphragm. This deep breathing, known as diaphragmatic breathing, enhances oxygen intake and supports a calm, focused state of mind.

Seated Sun Salutations: A Complete Sequence

Sun Salutations, or Surya Namaskar, are a series of poses performed in a flow, traditionally used to warm up the body. In chair yoga, we adapt this sequence to be performed while seated.

- **Seated Mountain Pose:** Begin in a seated mountain pose, sitting erect with your feet flat on the floor. Your hands rest on your thighs.

- **Raised Arms Pose:** Inhale and lift your arms up overhead, palms facing each other.

- **Seated Forward Bend:** Exhale and gently fold forward from your hips, lowering your hands towards your feet. Keep your spine straight.

- **Halfway Lift:** Inhale and lift your body halfway up, with your hands on your knees and your back flat.

- **Return to Seated Mountain Pose:** Exhale and gently fold forward again. Then inhale, lifting your arms back overhead, and return to the seated mountain pose.

Repeat this sequence 5-10 times, coordinating each movement with your breath.

Flow Between Twists and Side Bends

This sequence integrates spinal twists and side bends, targeting the core, enhancing flexibility, and improving digestion.

- **Seated Spinal Twist:** From the seated mountain pose, inhale and as you exhale, twist to the right, placing your left hand on your right knee and your right hand behind you for support. Inhale back to center.

- **Seated Side Bend:** Inhale and lift your right arm up, bending to the left. Keep your left hand on your left thigh for support. Exhale back to center.

- **Repeat on the Opposite Side:** Repeat the twist and side bend on the opposite side.

Go through this sequence several times, flowing smoothly from one pose to the other.

Breath-Linked Core Series

Core strength is fundamental in yoga, and linking these movements with breath enhances their impact.

- **Seated Leg Lifts:** Sit at the edge of the chair. Inhale, and as you exhale, lift your right knee towards your chest. Inhale as you lower it. Repeat with the left leg.

- **Seated Bicycle:** Sit back slightly in your chair for support. Lift both feet off the ground and perform a bicycle pedaling motion, coordinating the movement with your breath.

- **Seated Side Twists:** Sit upright, extend your arms out to the sides at shoulder height. Twist to the right, reaching your left hand to the outside of your right knee. Inhale back to center, then exhale and twist to the left.

- Repeat each exercise for several rounds, keeping your movements slow and controlled.

Integrating Movement and Breath for a Full Chair Yoga Flow

A full chair yoga flow combines the sequences mentioned above into a cohesive practice. Begin with seated sun salutations to warm up the body, then transition into the flow between twists and side bends, and conclude with the breath-linked core series.

Throughout the flow, maintain a focus on your breath. Allow the breath to guide your movements, inhaling to expand or extend, and exhaling to contract or twist. This integration of movement and breath not only enhances physical benefits but also fosters a meditative state, reducing stress and promoting mental clarity.

CHAPTER 3

SPECIALIZED PRACTICES AND MODIFICATIONS

Adapting Chair Yoga for Different Fitness Levels

Understanding Individual Needs

The first step in adapting chair yoga is to assess and understand individual fitness levels. This assessment can take into account factors such as age, mobility, flexibility, and any pre-existing health conditions. Knowing your starting point helps in tailoring the yoga practice to suit your needs, ensuring that the exercises are both effective and safe.

Modifications for Beginners

For beginners, especially those who may have limited mobility or are new to exercise, the focus should be on gentle movements and basic poses. Modifications can include:

Shortening the duration of each pose.

- Using props like cushions for additional support.
- Reducing the range of motion in twists and stretches.

- Incorporating more guided relaxation and breathing exercises to build stamina gently.

Intermediate Adaptations

As you become more comfortable with the basics, you can gradually introduce more challenging poses and sequences. For intermediate practitioners, adaptations might include:

- Increasing the holding time for each pose.
- Introducing mild twists and forward bends to enhance flexibility.
- Incorporating standing poses using the chair for support, to build balance and strength.

Advanced Modifications

For those at an advanced fitness level, chair yoga can still be challenging and rewarding. Advanced modifications can involve:

- Integrating dynamic movements and flows between poses.
- Using the chair for more challenging balance poses.

- Adding light weights or resistance bands for strength training.

Chair Yoga for Improved Digestion and Metabolism

Yoga and Digestive Health

The digestive system is a complex mechanism that not only processes food but is also crucial for overall health and well-being. Yoga's holistic approach, which includes physical movements, breath control, and mental relaxation, can significantly impact digestive health. The physical movements help stimulate the gastrointestinal tract, the breathwork enhances oxygen flow to digestive organs, and the relaxation techniques reduce stress, which is often a contributing factor to digestive problems.

Physiological Effects

Yoga poses can increase blood circulation to the digestive organs, which helps in the efficient absorption of nutrients and the elimination of waste. Furthermore, the gentle pressure and stretching involved in certain yoga poses can aid in massaging internal organs, promoting movement and function.

Psychological Benefits

Stress is known to have a detrimental effect on digestion. Yoga's mindfulness and relaxation aspects play a key role in reducing stress and its impact on the gastrointestinal system. By lowering stress levels, yoga can help alleviate issues like irritable bowel syndrome (IBS) and acid reflux.

Targeted Poses for Digestion

Chair yoga includes several poses specifically beneficial for digestion. These poses are designed to be gentle yet effective, making them accessible for seniors or those with physical limitations.

Seated Spinal Twists

Twisting poses are excellent for stimulating digestion. A seated spinal twist involves rotating the torso, which can massage the abdominal organs and aid in the process of digestion and detoxification. This movement helps in stimulating peristalsis, the series of muscle contractions within the intestinal walls that moves food through the digestive system.

How to Perform:

- Sit upright in the chair, feet flat on the ground.
- Place your right hand on the left knee and your left hand behind you for support.
- Inhale deeply, elongating your spine.
- As you exhale, gently twist to the left. Hold for a few breaths.
- Return to center on an inhalation and repeat on the opposite side.

Forward Bends

Gentle forward bends can apply light pressure to the abdomen, which may help in stimulating the digestive organs. These movements can also be soothing for individuals experiencing bloating or gas.

How to Perform:

- Sit towards the front edge of the chair, feet flat on the ground.
- Inhale and raise your arms overhead.
- As you exhale, gently bend forward from your hips, lowering your hands towards your feet.

- Hold for a few breaths, then slowly rise back up on an inhalation.

Seated Side Bends

Side bends stretch and stimulate the sides of the body, including the liver and kidneys, essential organs for metabolism and detoxification.

How to Perform:

- Sit upright with your feet firmly planted on the ground.
- Raise your right arm towards the ceiling.
- On an exhale, gently bend to the left, keeping your right arm extended. Your left hand can rest on your left thigh for support.
- Hold for a few breaths, then return to the center and repeat on the other side.

Breathing Techniques

Pranayama, or yogic breathing, is an integral part of yoga that has profound effects on the body and mind, including digestive health.

1. Deep Abdominal Breathing

This breathing technique encourages full oxygen exchange and is beneficial for stimulating the digestive organs.

How to Practice:

- Sit comfortably in your chair, hands resting on your abdomen.
- Slowly inhale through your nose, feeling your abdomen expand under your hands.
- Exhale slowly through the nose, feeling the abdomen contract.
- Continue this deep, rhythmic breathing for several minutes.

2. Alternate Nostril Breathing

Alternate nostril breathing is known to balance the body's systems, including the digestive system, and can help in managing stress.

How to Practice:

- Sit comfortably with your back straight.
- Place your left hand on your lap and your right hand in front of your face.

- Close your right nostril with your thumb and inhale slowly through the left nostril.
- Close the left nostril with your ring finger, open the right nostril, and exhale.
- Inhale through the right nostril, close it, and exhale through the left.
- Continue this alternating pattern for several minutes.

Integrating Practices into Daily Life

To reap the full benefits of these chair yoga practices for digestion and metabolism, it's important to integrate them into your daily routine. Consistency is key. Even a few minutes of targeted chair yoga each day can make a significant difference in digestive health and overall well-being.

Balancing Exercises for Stability and Core Strength in Chair Yoga

Importance of Balance and Core Strength

For seniors and individuals with mobility issues, maintaining and improving balance and core strength is not just about fitness; it's a key aspect of their safety and independence. Falls are a leading cause of injury among older adults, and a strong core and good balance are essential defenses against this risk. Chair yoga emerges as a gentle yet effective way to cultivate these crucial abilities, providing a means to enhance physical stability and overall well-being in a safe, accessible manner.

Core-Strengthening Poses in Chair Yoga

The core muscles, including the abdominals, lower back, hips, and pelvis, play a vital role in maintaining balance and stability. Strengthening these muscles is a central aspect of chair yoga.

1. Seated Mountain Pose

- **Execution:** Sit upright in the chair with feet flat on the ground, aligning your head, shoulders, and hips. Engage your abdominal muscles by drawing them in towards your spine.
- **Benefits:** This pose strengthens the abdominal muscles and improves posture, which is fundamental for balance.

2. Chair Plank

- **Execution:** Sit at the edge of the chair, place your hands on the seat on either side of your hips, and stretch your legs forward. Engage your core and lift your hips, creating a straight line from your shoulders to your heels.

- **Benefits:** This pose targets the entire core region, including the abdominals, lower back, and shoulders, enhancing overall stability.

3. Seated Leg Lifts

- **Execution:** Sit upright and lift one leg at a time, keeping it straight, or bent if that's more comfortable. Hold the position briefly before lowering the leg.
- **Benefits:** This exercise strengthens the hip flexors and lower abdominals, key muscles for maintaining balance.

Balance-Enhancing Practices in Chair Yoga

Balance exercises in chair yoga can be adapted to suit various fitness levels, from beginners to more advanced practitioners.

1. Seated Tree Pose

- **Execution:** While seated, place the sole of one foot on the inner thigh or calf of the opposite leg, avoiding the knee joint. Raise your arms overhead or keep them in a prayer position.

- **Benefits:** This pose enhances focus and stability, engaging the core muscles for balance.

2. Standing Poses Using the Chair

- **Execution:** Use the chair for support while practicing standing poses like Warrior or Half-Moon. The chair provides stability as you work on your balance.
- **Benefits:** These poses improve leg strength, flexibility, and balance.

Dynamic Movements for Agility

Incorporating dynamic movements into chair yoga routines can significantly improve agility, coordination, and reaction time, all of which are crucial for preventing falls and enhancing mobility.

1. Arm Lifts and Twists

- **Execution:** While seated, lift your arms alternately or twist your torso, coordinating the movements with your breath.
- **Benefits:** These movements enhance upper body agility and coordination, aiding in overall balance.

2. Chair Sun Salutations

- **Execution:** Perform a modified version of the Sun Salutation sequence while seated or using the chair for support.
- **Benefits:** This series of movements improves flexibility and coordination, vital for maintaining agility.

3. Seated Marching

- **Execution:** Lift your knees alternately as if marching in place while seated.
- **Benefits:** This exercise improves lower body strength and coordination, contributing to better balance.

Relaxation and Mindfulness in Chair Yoga

The practice of relaxation and mindfulness in chair yoga is fundamental for overall wellness. Stress and anxiety can negatively impact balance and cognitive function, making relaxation techniques an integral part of balance training.

1. Guided Relaxation

- **Execution:** Engage in guided relaxation sessions at the end of your yoga practice, focusing on releasing tension from each body part.
- **Benefits:** This technique promotes overall relaxation, reduces stress, and enhances mental clarity, supporting balance and stability.

2. Meditation and Mindful Breathing

- **Execution:** Practice meditation and mindful breathing exercises, focusing on the rhythm of your breath and clearing your mind.
- **Benefits:** These practices improve focus and mental steadiness, which are crucial for maintaining physical balance.

3. Visualization Techniques

- **Execution:** Use visualization techniques to imagine yourself performing poses with ease and stability.
- **Benefits:** Visualization can improve confidence and mental preparation for physical activities, enhancing balance and coordination.

CHAPTER 4

INTEGRATING CHAIR YOGA INTO DAILY LIFE

Daily Short Practices for Consistent Results

The Power of Routine

Consistency is the key when it comes to reaping the benefits of any yoga practice, including chair yoga. Incorporating short chair yoga sessions into your daily routine can lead to significant improvements in flexibility, strength, and mental clarity. The beauty of chair yoga is its accessibility; you don't need a large space or an extended period. Even a few minutes can be beneficial.

Morning Rituals

Starting your day with a series of gentle chair yoga stretches can awaken your body and prepare your mind for the day ahead. Simple movements like neck rolls, shoulder shrugs, and spinal twists can be done right at your breakfast table. This not only loosens up the muscles but also stimulates blood flow and digestion.

Midday Movement Breaks

Incorporate chair yoga into your midday routine to combat the lethargy that often hits after lunch. A five-minute session comprising seated cat-cow stretches, side bends, and forward folds can re-energize you. This not only helps in maintaining physical flexibility but also serves as a mental reset, enhancing focus and productivity for the rest of the day.

Evening Wind-Down

Evenings are a great time for more introspective and calming chair yoga practices. Focus on longer holds and deep breathing to release the tensions of the day. Postures like the seated forward bend or gentle twists can aid in digestion and relaxation, preparing your body and mind for a restful night's sleep.

Mindful Eating and Chair Yoga: A Holistic Approach

The Connection Between Yoga and Eating

Chair yoga, a gentle and adaptable form of yoga, offers more than just physical benefits; it serves as a portal to a more mindful and holistic way of living, including the way we approach our eating habits. Mindfulness, a core principle in yoga, is the practice of being fully present and engaged in the moment. This concept, deeply rooted in yoga philosophy, extends beyond the yoga mat and can profoundly influence our relationship with food.

The Philosophy of Mindfulness in Yoga

Yoga teaches us to be aware of our body, our breath, and our thoughts. This awareness fosters a deeper connection with ourselves, enabling us to recognize and respond to our body's true needs. Applying this mindfulness to eating means being fully present during meals, paying attention to the tastes, textures, and smells of our food, and listening to our body's hunger and fullness cues.

Mindful Eating Practices

1. *Starting with Gratitude and Breathing*

Beginning a meal with a moment of gratitude or a short breathing exercise can transform the dining experience. This practice, borrowed from yoga, sets a tone of mindfulness. It helps us to pause, reflect, and appreciate the nourishment we are about to receive. This simple act of pausing can also shift our nervous system from a state of 'fight or flight' to a more relaxed 'rest and digest' mode, enhancing the digestive process.

2. Eating Slowly and Mindfully

Eating slowly and chewing thoroughly are essential aspects of mindful eating. This practice allows us to savor each bite and be more attuned to our body's signals of hunger and satiety. It can also prevent overeating and improve digestion, as the process of digestion begins in the mouth with the act of chewing.

3. The Experience of Savoring

Taking time to really taste our food heightens the dining experience. It encourages us to be present with the flavors and textures in our mouth, turning eating from a passive activity into an engaging sensory experience. This heightened awareness can lead to greater satisfaction with meals, often resulting in smaller portion sizes being consumed.

Aligning Food Choices with Yoga Principles

1. Awareness and Respect for the Body

Yoga instills a sense of awareness and respect for the body. This awareness can inspire healthier food choices that are more aligned with the body's needs. By listening to our body and understanding its needs, we can choose foods that nourish and energize us, rather than those that merely satisfy a momentary craving.

2. A Nourishing Diet

A diet that complements chair yoga practice is rich in nutrients and light on the digestive system. Fruits, vegetables, whole grains, and lean proteins provide the necessary nutrients without overburdening the body. These foods not only nourish the body but also support the energy and flexibility required for yoga practice.

3. The Importance of Hydration

Hydration plays a crucial role in our overall well-being and is an essential part of a mindful eating routine. Drinking plenty of water throughout the day aids digestion, keeps the body's systems functioning optimally, and helps maintain energy levels. In yoga, water is often seen as a cleansing agent, flushing toxins from the body and clearing the mind.

Deepening Mindful Eating through Chair Yoga Practice

1. *Yoga Postures to Enhance Digestion*

Certain chair yoga postures are specifically beneficial for digestion. Gentle twists, forward bends, and stretches can stimulate the digestive organs, promoting better digestion and alleviating discomfort. These movements can be integrated before or after meals to support the digestive process.

2. *Breathing Techniques for Mindful Eating*

Pranayama, or yogic breathing techniques, can also support mindful eating. Practices like diaphragmatic breathing help in calming the mind and preparing the body for a relaxed eating experience. This relaxed state allows for better digestion and a more mindful approach to eating.

3. *Meditation and Mindfulness*

Meditation, another key element of yoga, enhances our capacity for mindfulness, which can be directly applied to eating habits. Regular meditation practice cultivates an inner sense of calm and presence, qualities that are essential for mindful eating.

The Synergy of Chair Yoga and Mindful Eating

1. *Holistic Health and Well-being*

The combination of chair yoga and mindful eating addresses health and well-being from a holistic perspective. While chair yoga strengthens and tones the body, mindful eating nourishes and respects it. Together, they create a balanced approach to health that encompasses physical, mental, and emotional well-being.

2. *Consistency and Routine*

Establishing a routine that incorporates both chair yoga and mindful eating can lead to more consistent health benefits. Just as chair yoga becomes more effective with regular practice, mindful eating habits become more ingrained and beneficial when practiced consistently.

3. *Transformative Lifestyle Changes*

Integrating chair yoga and mindful eating into daily life can lead to transformative lifestyle changes. This holistic approach encourages a more connected and harmonious way of living, where food is not just fuel but a source of nourishment for both the body and soul.

Stress Management: Relaxation and Meditation Techniques

Understanding Stress and Yoga

In our fast-paced world, stress is a common experience, yet its impact on our health and well-being can be profound. Chronic stress can lead to a range of health issues, including weight gain, sleep disturbances, anxiety, and a weakened immune system. Yoga, especially chair yoga, offers a viable solution for managing stress. It combines physical postures with relaxation and meditation techniques to create a holistic approach to stress reduction.

The Foundations of Stress Reduction in Yoga

Yoga addresses stress by promoting a sense of harmony and balance in both the body and mind. Chair yoga, with its gentle approach, is particularly suitable for those who may find traditional yoga practices physically challenging. It focuses on releasing tension, enhancing breath control, and fostering a state of mindful awareness.

Breathing Exercises (Pranayama)

Pranayama, or yogic breathing, is a cornerstone of stress management in yoga. These techniques help regulate the nervous system, shift the body's balance from the stress-induced "fight or flight" response to a more relaxed "rest and digest" state. Let's delve into some effective pranayama techniques:

- **Diaphragmatic Breathing:** This involves deep breathing into the belly, which helps activate the parasympathetic nervous system, responsible for relaxation. Practicing diaphragmatic breathing can lower heart rate and blood pressure, inducing a state of calm.

- **Alternate Nostril Breathing (Nadi Shodhana):** This technique involves alternating the breath through each nostril. It helps balance the left and right hemispheres of the brain, creating a sense of equilibrium and mental clarity.

- **Bhramari (Bee Breath):** This involves making a humming sound during exhalation. It's known for its ability to soothe the mind and reduce anxiety.

Meditation and Mindfulness Practices

Chair yoga seamlessly integrates meditation and mindfulness practices, crucial for managing stress. These practices involve focusing the mind and creating a sense of presence, which helps in breaking the cycle of chronic stress and anxiety.

- **Focused Breath Meditation:** This involves concentrating on the breath, bringing attention back whenever the mind wanders. This practice enhances mental focus and fosters a sense of inner peace.

- **Guided Imagery:** Here, you're guided to visualize calming and peaceful images. This technique is useful in reducing anxiety and promoting relaxation.

- **Body Scan Meditation:** This involves mentally scanning your body for areas of tension and consciously releasing it. It helps in developing awareness of bodily sensations and aids in relaxation.

Integrating Relaxation Techniques Throughout the Day

The beauty of chair yoga's relaxation techniques lies in their adaptability to everyday situations. They can be practiced almost anywhere, at any time, making them highly effective for managing daily stress.

- **Breathing Before Responding:** Taking a few deep breaths before responding in a stressful situation can help maintain a calm demeanor.

- **Mindfulness Breaks:** Practicing a few minutes of mindfulness during breaks at work or home can significantly lower stress levels and improve concentration.

- **Evening Relaxation Routine:** Engaging in a brief session of chair yoga or meditation before bed can promote better sleep quality and relaxation.

The Role of Restorative Chair Yoga Poses

Restorative chair yoga poses are specifically designed to promote relaxation and stress relief. These poses involve gentle stretching and are often held for longer periods, allowing the body to release tension.

- **Seated Forward Bend (Paschimottanasana):** This pose helps in calming the mind and relieving stress. It can be modified to be done while sitting on a chair.

- **Seated Cat-Cow Stretch:** This involves moving the spine from a rounded position (cat) to an arched one (cow). It's excellent for releasing back tension and promoting spinal flexibility.

- **Chair Pigeon Pose:** This pose, done while seated, helps in opening the hips, which is where we often store emotional stress.

- **Seated Twist (Ardha Matsyendrasana):** Twists are known for their ability to rejuvenate and relax. A gentle seated twist can aid in digestion and release tension in the spine.

- **Seated Savasana:** Although traditionally done lying down, Savasana can be adapted for the chair. It involves sitting comfortably, closing the eyes, and focusing on relaxation and breath, allowing the body and mind to completely relax.

CHAPTER 5

PROGRESSING IN YOUR CHAIR YOGA JOURNEY

Tracking Your Progress: Tips and Tricks

Set Clear, Achievable Goals: Begin by setting specific, measurable, achievable, relevant, and time-bound (SMART) goals. These could range from improving flexibility and balance to reducing stress or belly fat.

Keep a Yoga Journal: Documenting your journey in a journal can be incredibly rewarding. Note down the poses you practice, the duration of each session, and any feelings or sensations you experience. This not only tracks your progress but also helps in understanding how your body and mind respond to different practices.

Regular Check-Ins: Schedule weekly or monthly check-ins with yourself. Reflect on your goals, what you've achieved, and what challenges you've faced. This regular assessment can provide insight into areas needing more focus.

Photographic or Video Documentation: Sometimes, visual evidence of your progress can be very motivating.

Taking photos or videos periodically can show changes in your posture, flexibility, and possibly physical appearance over time.

Seek Feedback: If you attend a class or have a coach, regularly ask for feedback. Understanding an external perspective can provide insights into improvements and areas for further development.

Celebrate Milestones: Recognize and celebrate your achievements, no matter how small. This positive reinforcement can boost your morale and keep you motivated.

Advanced Chair Yoga Poses for Further Development

1. Chair Pigeon Pose (Eka Pada Rajakapotasana)

This pose is excellent for opening the hips and improving lower body flexibility, which is crucial for maintaining mobility and balance.

- **How to Perform:** Sit upright in your chair with feet flat on the ground. Lift your right ankle and place it over your left knee, creating a figure-four shape.

Gently lean forward from the hips, maintaining a straight back. Hold this position while taking deep breaths, then switch legs.

- **Benefits:** Increases hip flexibility, reduces lower back strain, and can alleviate sciatic pain.
- **Modifications:** If leaning forward is challenging, simply sitting upright while maintaining the figure-four leg position can also be beneficial.

2. Twisted Chair Pose (Parivrtta Utkatasana)

This pose involves a gentle twist, which is great for the torso, aiding digestion, and working the obliques.

- **How to Perform:** Sit sideways on your chair. Keeping your feet flat on the floor, twist your torso towards the back of the chair, holding the backrest for support. Ensure your spine is elongated during the twist. Repeat on the other side.
- **Benefits:** Enhances spinal mobility, stimulates digestion, and tones the abdominal muscles.
- **Modifications:** For a less intense twist, don't use the backrest for support; instead, twist using your core strength.

3. Chair Warrior III (Virabhadrasana III)

This is a balancing pose that strengthens the core and improves focus.

- **How to Perform:** Stand behind the chair, holding onto the backrest. Extend one leg backward while leaning your torso forward, forming a 'T' shape with your body. Keep your extended leg and spine in a straight line. Hold this position, then switch legs.
- **Benefits:** Strengthens the core, legs, and arms; improves balance and concentration.
- **Modifications:** Keep the supporting leg slightly bent if needed, or perform the pose without holding onto the chair for more challenge.

4. Chair Extended Side Angle (Utthita Parsvakonasana)

This pose stretches the waist and strengthens the side muscles, enhancing lateral flexibility.

- **How to Perform:** Sit on the chair with feet flat on the floor. Extend one arm overhead while bending your torso to the opposite side, keeping your other hand on your thigh. Stretch as far as comfortable, then switch sides.

- **Benefits:** Stretches and strengthens the side muscles, improves flexibility of the spine, and aids in breathing capacity.
- **Modifications:** For a deeper stretch, slide your lower hand down the outside of your leg.

5. Chair Eagle Pose (Garudasana)

A pose that challenges balance and coordination, this is ideal for improving joint mobility.

- **How to Perform:** Sit upright and cross one thigh over the other, hooking your foot behind the lower leg if possible. Stretch your arms forward, crossing them at the elbows, and intertwine your wrists. Hold this pose with a straight back, then unravel and switch sides.
- **Benefits:** Enhances joint mobility in the arms and legs, improves balance and concentration.
- **Modifications:** If entwining the legs is difficult, simply cross them at the knees without hooking the foot.

6. Seated Forward Bend (Paschimottanasana)

This pose is excellent for stretching the hamstrings and lower back, promoting flexibility and relieving tension.

- **How to Perform:** Sit with legs extended forward and spine straight. Hinge at the hips and lean forward, reaching towards your toes. Keep the back straight and only bend as far as comfortable.
- **Benefits:** Stretches the hamstrings and lower back, promotes inner thigh flexibility, and can calm the mind.
- **Modifications:** Bend your knees slightly if the stretch is too intense, or use a yoga strap around your feet to aid the forward bend.

Incorporating Breathing and Mindfulness

While practicing these poses, it's important to focus on your breath. Breathe deeply and evenly, using the breath to guide your movements. This not only enhances the physical benefits of each pose but also brings a mindfulness aspect to your practice, helping you stay connected and present.

Listening to Your Body

Remember, the goal of yoga is not to push your body into uncomfortable positions but to find a balance between challenge and ease. Listen to your body's signals and modify each pose to suit your current level of flexibility and strength. It's about progress, not perfection.

Regular Practice

Consistency is key in advancing your chair yoga journey. Aim to practice regularly, even if it's just for a few minutes a day. Over time, you will notice improvements in your flexibility, strength, and overall well-being.

Staying Motivated: Building a Sustainable Routine

Maintaining motivation is crucial in any fitness journey, especially in practices like chair yoga, where the progress can be subtle and gradual. Building a sustainable routine requires a mix of discipline, self-awareness, and a positive mindset. Here's a deeper look into how you can stay motivated and make chair yoga an integral part of your life.

Variety in Practice

Variety is the spice of life, and this holds true for yoga practice as well. Varying your routines keeps them fresh and engaging, preventing monotony which can lead to a loss of interest.

- **Experiment with Different Poses:** Don't just stick to the same set of poses. Explore new ones, especially those that challenge different muscle groups. This not only enhances physical benefits but also keeps your mind actively engaged.

- **Alter Sequences and Duration:** Change the order of poses and the length of your practice. Some days, you might focus on a longer, more meditative session, while other days could be about quick, energizing flows.

- **Theme Your Sessions:** Having themes, like balance, flexibility, or strength, can give each session a purpose and make your practice more goal-oriented.

Set a Regular Schedule

Consistency in practice is key to seeing results and staying motivated.

- **Dedicate a Specific Time:** Choose a time of day when you feel most energetic and least likely to be disturbed. This could be early morning or a quiet time in the afternoon.

- **Make it a Ritual:** Treat your yoga time as a non-negotiable appointment. Setting it as a recurring event in your calendar can be a helpful reminder.

- **Prepare Your Space in Advance:** Have your chair, mat, and any other accessories ready. This removes barriers to starting your session and helps in building a routine.

Join a Community

Being part of a yoga community can provide invaluable support.

- **Local Classes or Groups:** Joining a local chair yoga class can provide a sense of camaraderie. Sharing the space with others who have similar goals can be highly motivating.

- **Online Communities:** If attending in-person classes isn't feasible, online forums or virtual classes can be equally beneficial. Engaging in discussions, sharing experiences, and receiving feedback can keep you motivated.

- **Participate in Events:** Be it virtual workshops or community yoga events, participating in these activities can enhance your connection to the practice and the community.

Incorporate Mindfulness and Meditation

Chair yoga is not just a physical practice; it's a holistic approach to wellness.

- **Start or End with Meditation:** Incorporate a few minutes of meditation at the beginning or end of your yoga practice. This helps in centering your mind, reducing stress, and enhancing the overall experience.

- **Practice Mindful Breathing:** Pay attention to your breath during practice. This mindfulness aspect can transform the experience, turning it into a meditative activity.

- **Body Scan Relaxation:** Occasionally, replace physical practice with a mindfulness exercise like a body scan. This promotes mental relaxation and body awareness.

Educate Yourself

Continuous learning keeps the mind engaged and the practice evolving.

- **Read Books and Articles:** Dive into literature about yoga, its history, and its health benefits. Understanding the 'why' behind your practice can be incredibly motivating.

- **Watch Documentaries or Listen to Podcasts:** Expand your knowledge through different media. Learning about others' experiences and insights can provide new perspectives.

- **Attend Workshops or Seminars:** These can be invaluable for deepening your understanding and refreshing your motivation.

Listen to Your Body

Attuning to your body's needs and limitations is crucial.

- **Understand Your Limits:** Acknowledge that some days you may need a gentler practice. Respect your body's signals to avoid over-exertion.

- **Modify Poses as Needed:** Use props or adapt poses to suit your comfort level. This individualization makes the practice sustainable.

- **Monitor Physical Responses:** Be aware of how your body feels during and after practice. This helps in fine-tuning your routine for optimal benefits.

Find an Accountability Partner

An accountability partner can be a powerful motivator.

- **Choose Someone with Similar Goals:** Partner with a friend or family member who is also interested in yoga or wellness. Sharing the journey can be mutually beneficial.

- **Regular Check-Ins:** Have regular sessions or conversations with your partner about your progress, challenges, and experiences.

- **Encourage and Support Each Other:** Celebrate each other's successes and offer support during setbacks.

Reward Yourself

Acknowledging your efforts and achievements can boost your motivation.

- **Set Milestones and Rewards:** Create small milestones in your practice and associate them with rewards like a special treat, a new yoga accessory, or a relaxing activity.

- **Non-Material Rewards:** Rewards don't always have to be tangible. A self-care day or an extra hour of sleep can be equally gratifying.

- **Visualize the Rewards:** Sometimes, just visualizing the reward can be a motivator in itself.

Reflect on the Benefits

Regular reflection on the positive changes brought about by your practice can reinforce your commitment.

- **Keep a Progress Diary:** Write down not just your physical progress but also any mental or emotional changes you observe.

- **Share Your Journey:** Sometimes, sharing your progress with others can make you more aware of how far you've come.

- **Acknowledge the Non-Physical Benefits:** Improvements in mood, stress levels, or sleep quality are as significant as physical changes and deserve recognition.

Embrace Challenges

Facing and overcoming challenges is part of the growth process.

- **View Challenges as Learning Opportunities:** Each challenge is a chance to learn something new about yourself and your practice.

- **Set Challenging, Yet Achievable Goals:** Push your boundaries, but do so in a realistic and safe manner.

- **Celebrate Overcoming Obstacles:** Acknowledge your resilience and strength in facing challenges. This not only boosts confidence but also reinforces your commitment to the practice.

CONCLUSION

In concluding this book, we reflect on the enriching journey of chair yoga for seniors, a journey that intertwines the gentle discipline of physical exercise with the nurturing embrace of mindfulness. This book has been an exploration into how chair yoga serves not just as a form of physical activity, but as a holistic approach to wellness, especially tailored for the unique needs of seniors.

Through the pages of this book, we have seen how chair yoga stands as a beacon of accessibility and adaptability, offering an effective way for seniors to enhance their physical health and combat belly fat, while simultaneously nurturing their mental and emotional well-being. The physical benefits of chair yoga, such as improved flexibility, strengthened muscles, and enhanced mobility, address the key concerns of aging, promoting a lifestyle that is both active and balanced.

We delved into the importance of adapting yoga practices to individual needs, emphasizing the significance of choosing the right equipment and modifying poses for safety and comfort. This adaptation is not just about physical adjustments; it's about cultivating a deeper awareness of one's body, listening to its signals, and respecting its limitations, thereby enhancing the personal yoga journey.

The theme of building a sustainable practice has been central to our discussion. We explored various strategies to maintain motivation in practicing chair yoga, from setting a regular schedule and incorporating variety to being part of a community. The role of mindfulness and meditation was highlighted, underscoring that chair yoga transcends physical benefits, touching upon mental serenity and emotional equilibrium.

Moreover, we emphasized the importance of embracing challenges as opportunities for growth and learning. The journey through chair yoga is not without its obstacles, but facing and overcoming these challenges is part of what makes this practice so fulfilling and empowering.

As we close this book, we hope that the insights and guidance provided here will inspire seniors to embark on or continue their chair yoga journey with renewed enthusiasm and dedication. Chair yoga is more than just an exercise; it's a path to a healthier, more balanced, and fulfilling lifestyle, offering a harmonious blend of physical activity, mental clarity, and emotional wellness. May this book serve as a companion and guide on your journey towards a life of greater health, vitality, and joy.